ROWING MADE SIMPLE: A Step-by-Step Guide to Mastering Workouts as a Beginner

Kendra Raymond

Table of Contents

CHAPTER ONE

INTRODUCTION

Right when you start another movement plan the essential thing that hits home is definitively accurate thing kind of action will be the most helpful and is it something that you will remain with. Rowing is an unprecedented all body practice and in addition to that, it's great times! That staggering thing is that it figures out your entire body anyway not the least bit like high impact practices with a rowing working there is a for the most part protected of injury. The following are a piece of the surprising benefits of a rowing exercise:

1. Low impact - The improvement is required when you are playing out a rowing exercise if smooth and recognizable. Since there are no unexpected impacts there is less bet of injury. If you keep your improvements a rival rhythm the strain on your joints, is insignificant not typical for a few unique exercises.

2. It works fundamentally every body part - Various activities don't offer the extent of improvement that a rowing exercise does. Locales, for instance, the upper arms, shoulders and back that get missed in various activities you will find with consistent exercise center schedules begin to take on a nice drawing in structure.

3. Extraordinary calorie burner - The way that rowing takes in a colossal number of muscle bundles makes it an eminent calorie burner. In case you show up for an hour at a searing pace you can wreck to 800 calories.

4. Increase mass - notwithstanding the way that paddling is an exceptional calorie consuming activity it's a dumbfounding technique for getting mass. The best part is that as you gain mass with each exercise you consume considerably more calories per meeting.

5. Inconceivable for extending genuine perseverance - As you happen with consistent work-out schedules you will see that you can practice for longer ranges.

Each gathering chips away at your cardiovascular prosperity. The better your cardiovascular prosperity is the more capable your body becomes at consuming fat.

6. There are various phenomenal work-out plans open - Online offers numerous unbelievable rec center routine timetables for line machines, it simply requires several snapshots of web examining to go over heaps of them. Like some other movement ensure when an activity you need to go through the commonplace broadening plan. While rowing is low impact your body really ought to be warmed up and chilled off. While starting your rowing routine progressively start until you achieve the best power. While

completing a gathering consistently postponed down to a stop. These are crucial advances which numerous people will frequently disregard.

This genuinely is an astonishing all body works out. Your legs, arms and center need to work in a condition of concordance consuming calories and getting mass. As you become more grounded you can increase your activity by adding block. As you add block you understand you're pushing your body impeccably. As referred to in advance rowing is heaps of silliness. Rowing machines that at in the activity habitats and, shockingly, the ones you can buy for your home rec focus are astonishing reenactments of certified water rowing.

GUIDELINES TO USE A ROWING MACHINE PROPERLY

The rowing machine is one of the health club's best machines yet several people use it since they don't see precisely exact thing a nice activity rowing is. Sorting out some way to use a rowing machine, comparable as swimming, gives an activity to your whole body! It is a staggering strategy for working your body, finish your cardio and consume a few hundred calories. Knowing this, could you verify or refute that you are more captivated to endeavor that elusive machine that you've been taking a gander at toward the side of the activity community? Time to tell yourself the best way to use a rowing machine!

This is the method for using a rowing machine: the key thing you will keep up with that ought to do after you plunk down is to try to change the foot lashes to meet your feet. Your effect focuses should incline gently against the underpinnings of the foot pedals and you truly need to guarantee that the foot tie is secure. If you are new to rowing, you should try to set the settings at a lower level (or the most negligible level in case you are totally new on the rowing machine). Once died down into the seat, you'll have to guarantee that your grip is firm and free. With these clear tips and you can tell yourself the best way to use a rowing machine. Methodology on the most ideal way to use a rowing machine implies a lot to the advancement of the activity. If your design isn't perfect, you could hurt your back. While rowing, you want to rely upon the muscles in your hips and legs to do by far most of the work. As you finish a stroke endeavor to evade unnecessarily bending your back. Sit upstanding and slant forward at your hips. Keep your elbows close to your body while you are pulling on the oars (or handles, dependent upon the kind of rowing machine you are using). You have now told yourself the best way to use a rowing machine congrats. There are three huge exercises that occur while sorting out some way to use a rowing machine and telling others the best way to use a rowing machine. The first is the stunt. The second is the power stroke and the third is known as the recovery. The catch is the place where you continue. Your knees should be bowed and held close to your body. Your chest region should lean forward fairly anyway your position shouldn't slacken. The power stroke is the name given to the development of you pushing on the foot pedals and widening your legs. All the while you bring your hands toward you. You truly need to inhale out during this development. At your body's most outrageous extension, lean back a touch, yet don't lean back unnecessarily far. This will guarantee your body gets the most possible benefit from the power stroke. Finally, the recovery is the place where you fix your arms, bend your knees and push your body ahead.

CHAPTER TWO

ROWING MACHINE WHY YOU SHOULD USE ONE

There are numerous inspirations driving why you should use a rowing machine. First of all, a rower is one of the most staggering pieces of stuff to grow your wellbeing, because not by any stretch like various types of movement machines, a rower outfits you with a full body practice which centers around different muscles in your body all the while. The muscles that are used when you play out a rowing exercise consolidate your back, your shoulders, your thighs, your arms, your strong strength, and fairly, your chest.

Another benefit of using rowing machines is that they give you a low impact practice which is essentially less troubling on your joints besides working your muscles a rower will increase cardiovascular wellbeing, work on the heart, and enable you to consume a lot of calories. The reality of the situation is that the more muscles you can use at any one given time will drive your body to consume more calories to complete what you are doing. Whether you want to lose some weight, work on your wellbeing, or tone your muscles, you will be competent show up at your targets with a rowing machine. It really is a securely of rec center hardware. There are numerous sorts of rowers accessible, and now and again figuring out which one you should get can be irksome. It on a very basic level depends upon what your goals are and how significant your pockets are. Rowing machines which rely upon a tension driven system are the most economical kind of rowers. At any rate this doesn't infer that they are not strong. I would concur that that in case you are a common person's who will probably either lose some weight, or further foster wellbeing levels, then, you should probably choose a strain driven rower, as it is more than gifted in helping you with showing up at your goals. On the contrary completion of the scale you get machines that use either air deterrent or water resistance. Such machines will commonly be more exorbitant, yet you genuinely get a lot of something different for your money. Such rowing machines are commonly used by people who need to take their health to much more raised level. It isn't really the situation that a complete juvenile cannot use one. A juvenile can staggering benefits from one of these machines, as well as someone who is more experienced, and these kinds of activity rowers will endure forever.

In the event that you are considering beginning some kind of work out regime or hoping to figure out, then, at that point, a paddling machine is an optimal decision. You will consume more calories by doing an obstruction paddling activity than you would do by utilizing an activity bicycle or a treadmill, basically in light of the fact that your body is compelled to utilize more muscle to play out an activity. Assuming you are unpracticed, you should see as your level first. This implies for the initial not many days do a few tests by perceiving how long you can push for before you begin feeling drained or running winded. Ensure that each time you practice on your rower, you record the time you spend working out, and the speed that you work out. Most rowers will have a presentation screen which will give you this data. When you sort out what amount of time it requires for you to begin feeling the speed, you have a beginning stage. For instance, on the off chance that you can at first column for 10 minutes, then the following time add 30-60 seconds to your paddling exercise. It may not seem like a ton, but rather it will all accumulate in the next few long stretches of time. You want to logically prepare. This implies adding a touch additional time each time you work out. Your body can adjust rapidly to what you do, so assuming you do a similar measure of activity at each exercise you won't get to the next level. By adding more in little advances you force your body to continue to adjust consistently. This implies better wellness, better muscle tone, and more consuming of calories. On the off chance that you were uncertain regarding the reason why you ought to utilize a paddling machine, then, at that point, ideally now you have a more clear thought. Essentially put there is next to no out there which can match what a paddling machine can offer you.

INDOOR PADDLING MACHINE TYPES EVALUATED

With paddling a very much perceived high advantage low effect exercise, there has been a major development in the kind and measure of indoor paddling machines available. It is critical to comprehend the various kinds and which might be fit best to your own insight and requirements prior to putting resources into one. Paddling is turning into an undeniably famous activity because of the way that it gives both high-impact molding and strength preparing. Utilizing an indoor paddling machine is a low effect exercise as far as weight on joints because of its perfection, while as yet conveying high effect results as all significant muscle bunches are being worked out. Various pieces of the body, for example, back shoulder, thigh and arm muscles are reinforced while utilizing an indoor rower, as well as your heart and lungs getting an extraordinary exercise prompting expanded endurance. This settles on it a famous decision in exercise center offices as well as among wellness lovers.

There are 4 unique kinds of indoor paddling machines to pick between, all giving incredible exercises whether a beginner of expert rower. The sorts are characterized by the strategy in which they give protection from the paddling activity, or at the end of the day how they reproduce the obstruction you would get from water assuming that you were out on the lake paddling.

The main sort we will take a gander at is a water driven paddling machine which really utilizes safeguard game plans to give the protection from the client. The obstruction is regularly changed on the water driven chamber contingent upon how hard you need your exercise. Typically these are the least expensive choice of paddling machines accessible as many won't be guaranteed to reproduce the full movement of the paddling activity, for example, the leg drive. Anyway they actually give a brilliant exercise and, as the majority of them are very convenient, give an incredible arrangement in the event that you are space or cost obliged. The second kind of indoor paddling machine is the attractive paddling machine. As the name proposes, the opposition in these rowers is given by magnets, ordinarily neutralizing a flywheel to reproduce the water obstruction. These rowers are described by their quietness and perfection, prompting them being very well known among rowers. They take into account the full scope of paddling developments and keeping in mind that being more costly than most water driven rowers, actually are actually reasonable. Some of them are very conservative as well, however beginning with this sort of rower and with practically all the rower types we will take a gander at next, and they are transcendently not effortlessly put away and are hence best left set-up.

Likewise beginning at this level, the rowers will generally accompany some kind of screen or show intended to give criticism to the client on their exercise. This data incorporates things like the time and the distance covered, number of strokes taken, number of strokes each moment and numerous other helpful insights that the more serious rower can use to work on their presentation. Some of them additionally have inputs for pulse screens so the client can advance their exhibition as they exercise.

The third kind of indoor rower we will take a gander at is the air paddling machine. The air rowers were the top choices for serious and proficient rowers for a long time, and it is just with the appearance of the following sort of rower we will take a gander at presently that has seen some get away from these, yet and still, at the end of the day not totally. The obstruction in an air rower is given by the progression of air over a fan-wheel or flywheel. The extraordinary fascination of the air rowers to numerous serious rowers is that this arrangement of opposition is automatic in that as you increment the stroke rate, the sped up the flywheel makes more prominent obstruction, which is precisely exact thing you would encounter were you really paddling on untamed water. It is for this near genuine sensation of paddling experience that this sort of rower has turned into the most famous, both in exercise centers and in homes.

The activity on the air paddling machines is exceptionally smooth and consistent, and these rowers consider full leg drive and consistent with life paddling activities. They truly do produce a touch of commotion with the air going over the flywheel are they are not conservative. While some have simple delivery frameworks for speedy getting together, they actually take up a lot of room and are best left set up and prepared for the following exercise.

The fourth and last sort we will take a gander at is the water paddling machine. These are the latest kind to enter the paddling machine market and they are turning out to be progressively well known among serious rowers. Obstruction is given through a flywheel that has paddles joined in an encased polycarbonate tank of water to give opposition likewise to a paddle or oar through water. Similarly as with the air rowers, the opposition is automatic and extremely smooth, providing the client with a colossally sensible sensation of paddling. The water rowers are the most costly of the kinds, however a portion of the makers have perceived this, thus have fostered their units to be exceptionally sharp and very much created as they are probably going to be left set up more often than not as well.

With the advantages of paddling now very much valued by those searching for a low effect exercise yet at the same time with perfect results it is just normal there are numerous makers giving quality items into the market. Whether or not you are simply beginning or an exceptionally experienced rower, there are models out there which will address your issues more than sufficiently. Simply take as much time as necessary and figure out which ones are selling great inside every class, as these will ordinarily be the models the vast majority perceive as the most ideal decision for their own venture.

CHAPTER THREE

SHOW CYCLE AND LINE LIKE AN ACE

On the off chance that you're going to begin showing a class that incorporates both indoor cycling and indoor paddling, the following are a couple of tips. Remain off the bicycle. To deal with every one of the factors in a cycling/paddling class, you'll should be on your feet, moving around the room.

Will you warm up? On-bicycle extends won't work in a split class. Conclude whether you'll start with a full-class stretch and warm-up, or have the members deal with that all alone. Dynamic Disengagement Extending is the most productive in class it warms the body as you stretch however they all occupy preparing time. Pre-plan your phases of preparation. You'll require a particular and definite paddling exercise, alongside your arranged cycling exercise. They don't need to run equal. That is, a 6:00 level on the bicycle doesn't need to run in a state of harmony with a 6:00 stretch on the paddling ergo meter (erg). They can assuming you like. Feel the distinctions between the two exercises. It is frequently inflexibly coordinated to Column exercises. That makes them powerful and simple to signal. Yet, probably the most disagreeable cycling exercises I've at any point done were a basically a made by a teacher rower. His classes appeared to be made with a number cruncher and a slide rule (a what?). All things considered, use cycling exercises that are like the ones you run now. Then you can form your paddling exercises without distancing your riders.

Gear your music for the bicycles. It's less vital to match music to a paddling drill, so continue to deal with your music the manner in which you have been. There are special cases for the most part execution related however by and large this turns out as expected. Retain the means for setting the erg screen. Idea 2 Models D and E utilize an intricate strategy for setting time or distance. You'll need to sign it like clockwork. On the off chance that you change mid-exercise from time to separate, be ready to re-sign. Model:

"Press Select Exercise. Press New Exercise. Press Time periods. Try not to establish the point in time yet! Utilize the Back Bolt to return to the "tens" segment. Set that for 1. Presently utilize the Forward Bolt to get to the "ones" segment. Presently press the mark at the lower part of the screen. That extensive depiction sets the clock briefly span. Assuming that they set the "ones" segment first to 0, it will default to a programmed ":20" (20 seconds). That messes up everything, and you'll need to invest energy evolving it. Continuously prompt the rowers first. Suppose you've chosen to run the exercises in equal arrangement, which is more straightforward for you. Separate the gatherings on their hardware. Prompt the rowers while the riders roll their legs. Instruct the rowers during their warm-up (say its 10 minutes). Simple warm-up easy route: Have them press "Line". They line as trained and stop when the PC clock comes to 10:00. While they column, you run a 10-minute bicycle warm-up. Once the warm-up is finished, the riders roll and recuperate while you signal the paddling preparing and setting the screen. This approach adjusts the significant changes for the two gatherings. The spans will be of a similar length, yet what the gatherings do during the stretches can be as comparable or as various as you like. Make a course of events. Assuming you like performing multiple tasks, go ahead and make exercises that don't look like each other by any means. You might require some kind of course of events to follow what's going on. Assuming you're a bookkeeping sheet nerd, that approach will be a good time for you. Assuming you're ready to monitor two distinct exercises intellectually with no cheat-sheet only let it all out. A timetable could be only a fundamental log with 3 to 4 segments. Minutes (0:00 to 30:00) go in the left section, paddling drills in the following, the cycling exercise in the third segment, and maybe notes and prompts for you in the fourth section. Utilize a stopwatch. You'll check your watch and know precisely exact thing everybody ought to do out of the blue.

All of this arranging makes making do and changing much simpler. You have your arrangement, yet still feel prepared to change at whatever point time or conditions call for it.

At the 30-minute imprint, switch hardware. The change will require a couple of moments, so abbreviate the warm-up, however allow everybody an opportunity to acclimate the objective muscles to the new action for the last part of the class. Restart your watch and rehash the body of the preparation. On the off chance that you can figure out how to do all of this AND convey content practice physiology, procedure, and preparing reasoning - your classes will be connecting with and educational, and appeal to an expansive base.

BENEFIT FROM A PADDLING MACHINE EXERCISE

Is it true that you are contemplating beginning a paddling machine gym routine so you can get in shape? There are a ton of smart reasons that you ought to utilize one of these machines, and it is by a wide margin one of the most mind-blowing ways of getting a full body exercise. On the off chance that you are somebody who is searching for a method for getting in shape and need to acquire some strength simultaneously, then, at that point, you will need to ensure you are aware of a portion of the extraordinary advantages that you will actually want to get when you utilize a paddling machine. One extraordinary advantage you will actually want to get from utilizing one of the air paddling machines that are accessible is endurance. This is an extraordinary method for developing how much endurance you have which can consider you to go longer. You will find that when you increment how much endurance you have, your energy level will likewise increment. This implies you won't feel so drained and tired constantly. There are different advantages you will actually want to get too. Utilizing a paddling machine includes hitting the treadmill. That implies you will actually want to consume off a ton of calories relying upon the length of your exercise. Assuming that you are on a legitimate eating routine and you really do practice that consumes calories then you will actually want to get in shape therefore. Another incredible advantage is the complete body strength that you will actually want to develop while utilizing this exercise machine. The muscles in your arms will be impacted however you will likewise see your abs and different muscles beginning to straighten out too. You can get in shape as well as you will actually want to acquire strength while utilizing one of these activity machines. These are only a couple of the extraordinary advantages you will actually want to get when you start your paddling machine exercise. Whether you are attempting to develop your endurance, get in shape, or gain strength, you will actually want to get precisely exact thing you are searching for from this one of these exercise machines. On the off chance that you are searching for one for your home rec center, investigate the air paddling machines that are accessible and conclude which one will work the best for your gym routine daily schedule.

THE END

www.ingramcontent.com/pod-product-compliance
Lightning Source LLC
Chambersburg PA
CBHW070751260726
48660CB00007B/3067